THE BOOK OF
DJED

FABLES
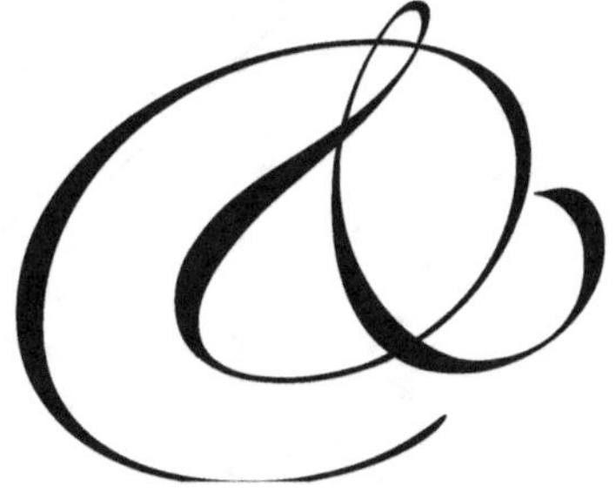
MYTHOLOGY

This book is dedicated to

NIKOERIK THE RED

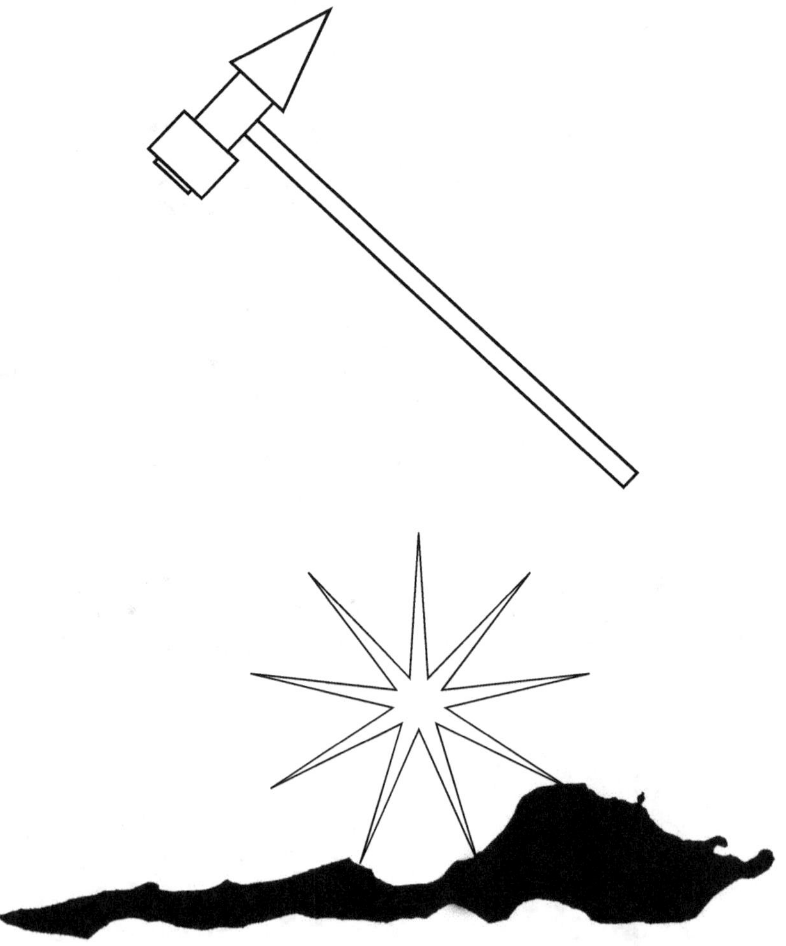

THE BOOK OF DJED

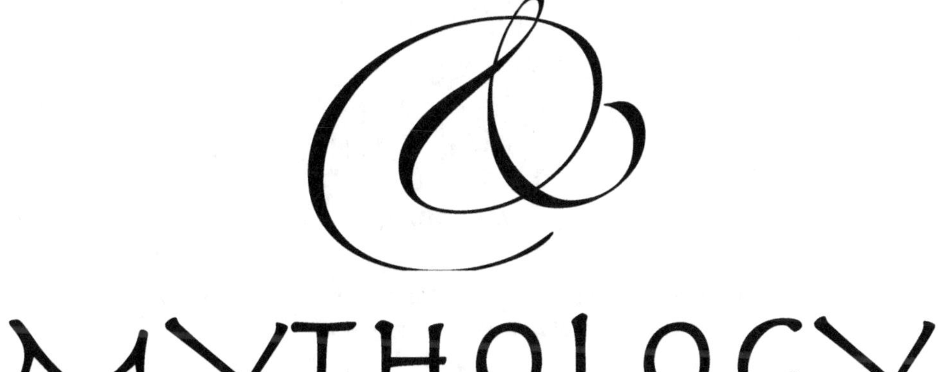

FABLES & MYTHOLOGY

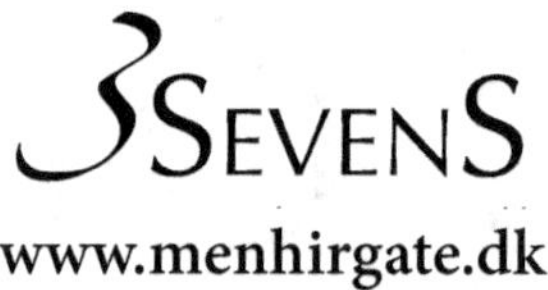

www.menhirgate.dk

Fremstilling og forlag: BoD – Books on Demand, Norderstedt, Tyskland
ISBN: 978-87-974199-4-6

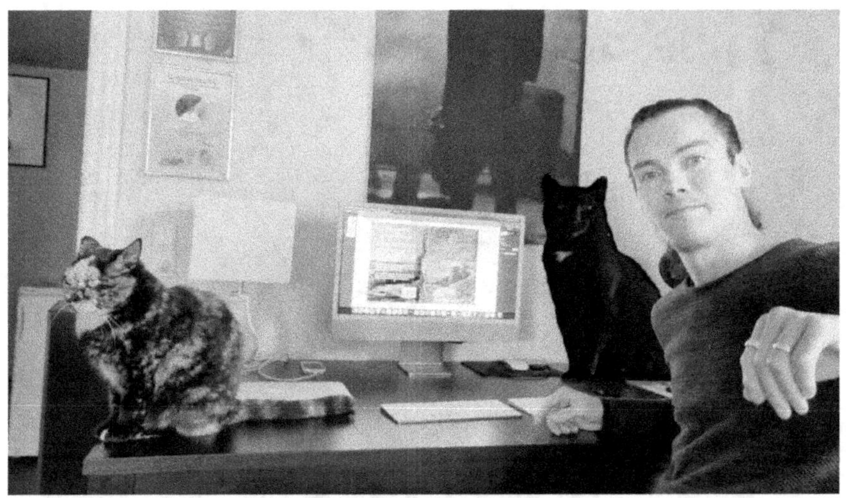

For 14 years, Jens Viktor Fraust has been researching natural healing, the psychology of personalities and spiritual, occult and mystical concepts, to find knowledge others can use to heal and improve themselves with.

Today he is a consultant specializing in creative problem solving, author of books and many health articles based on scientific publications. He is also a creator of documentaries and a lecturer.

He was originally trained in business school and later as an electrician, which proved to be an asset in understanding and explaining deep spiritual concepts based on electromagnetism. He is also a trained Gateway healer, Reiki healer and Regression therapist. In this book, Jens Viktor Fraust is Santa Claus himself who delivers gifts to you.

Table of Contents

THE LINEAGE

The name of my 600-year-old lineage is Thor, and originates from the place of Illumination surrounded by water in the northern seat of the kingdom of all countries in this world. Our purpose here is observation and information. We walk among you, we look like you, but we are the ones who save everyday life when your freedom is threatened. Only a being with the freedom to make its own choices is worth observing, therefore we cherish the freedom of all beings, which humans are unfortunately experts at trading away in fear. In the old days, Thor was another name for Düvel which means devil, and I am the devil as so many others are. The devil also called Satan in recent times and the number 666, along with today's horror movies scare people from finding the only way to healing and eternal life, and that is darkness. Darkness is turned into evil where the devil with the number 666 and the name Satan lives with the demons. Our real number is 9 and the symbol is a nine star. All living things are born out of the darkness, the great mother, and only that mother of darkness can heal and keep one alive forever. The mother of humanity is the dark, and therefore it is the dark that can heal almost anything, but you must have the courage to embrace the dark to find the light. We prefer to wear black or dark clothes and look after ourselves, but we help everyone who seeks shelter and healing with us. Human doctors and vets wear white coats and they are proven to have killed more humans and animals than the darkness ever has.

We work in the dark to serve the lighT

THE WORLD TREE

A tree's branches spread out into smaller and smaller branches and form the crown in the north. A tree's roots are branches like the tree's crown, just below the surface of the earth in the south. The top of the tree is called a crown just as kings and queens have a crown on their head. The word "world" comes from the word "whirl" which in Danish is used in the word "ryghvirvel" that means vertebra. The human spine is made of 33 vertebrae, and between them nerve pathways emerge that look like trees that branch out into smaller and smaller nerves to the parts of the body and back again to the spine. In the oldest and largest mythologies, the world is a metaphor for a human body, the world of one human being, that in religions are the garden with many trees. The world tree itself can be interpreted as the entire body's nervous system distributed via the spine. At the top of the spine is the crown, and at the base of the spine at the Cauda Equina begin the roots of the World Tree.

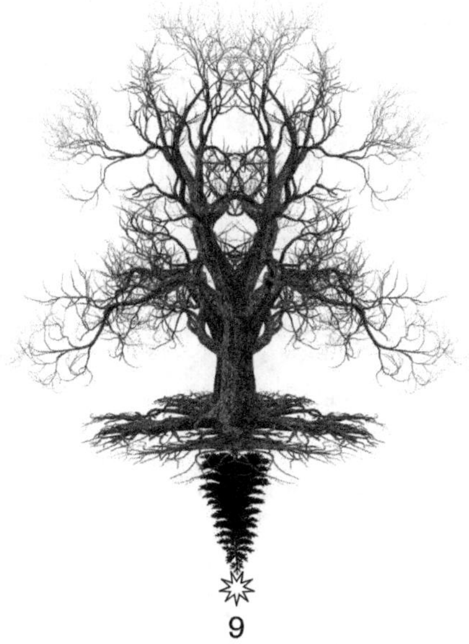

THE WATER THAT GIVES LIFE

In the brain there are two large ventricles called horns. There is a horn in the left and right hemisphere, they are the same size. Below these two horns is a third ventricle. These three ventricles convert blood into a salty liquid that tastes like metal. The liquid is suitable for conducting electric current. The fluid contains its own immune system of a special type of white blood cells. The liquid is called "Living water" or e.g. "Jordan River" or "mead". The liquid is personified as the man known as Jesus or John the Baptist. The name John comes from the word Iohn which is ion which in the old days was associated with water. The fluid's name today is cerebrospinal fluid, so now it is obviously true that John, baptize the body's nervous system in cerebrospinal fluid. The two high ventricles, and the third ventricle below them, are called Høj, Jævnhøj and Tredje in Norse mythology. In medical illustrations today, the words "horns" are used for the two large ventricles because they resemble horns, which are creator gods, for only with them can there be life in the body. In Norse mythology, the ventricles are also the deer Eiktyrnir, who from the roof of Valhalla eats the branches that are blood vessels, and turns them into cerebrospinal fluid that drips from the deer's horns down to the great fountain Hvergelmir.

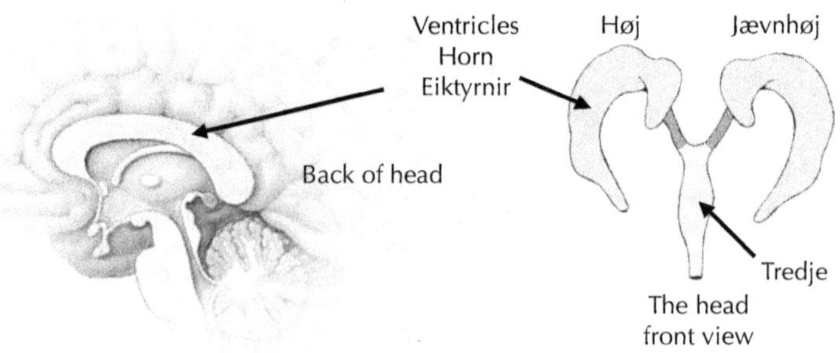

The gods, giants and heroes among the humans, also called Vikings, drink mead from horns, which is an analogy for the body's nervous system drinking mead from the horns in the brain. When the cerebrospinal fluid comes back after a long trip in the body's nervous system, it is actually more or less refined or simply stored and it is called "mead" that comes back to the creator gods Høj, Jævnhøj and Tredje who now drink a good round of refined mead.

THE KING AND THE QUEEN

The area of the brain called the third all-seeing eye has three major important areas. The first area is the king's room or seat and that is the pineal gland. Then there is the pituitary gland, the seat of the Queen. In the center of the third eye is the thalamus where all nerve pathways become 12 cranial nerve pathways from the left hemisphere and 12 cranial nerve pathways from the right hemisphere, a total of 24 cranial nerve pathways meet in the thalamus which is where you sense this life and from where you command the body. The 24 nerve pathways are the 24 elders in the Bible story.

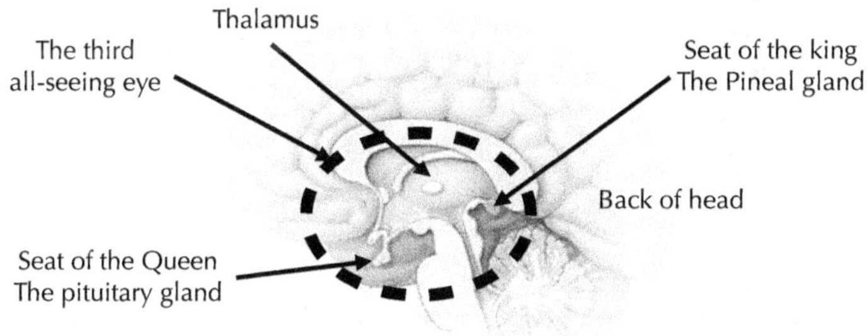

In Egypt, the right part of the thalamus is called the "Eye of Horus" which is the reception of senses. The left part of the thalamus is called the "Eye of Ra" which is one's extroverted actions. Horus is the moon which is the inner mind, introverted silence. Ra is the sun god and the sun is extroverted action.

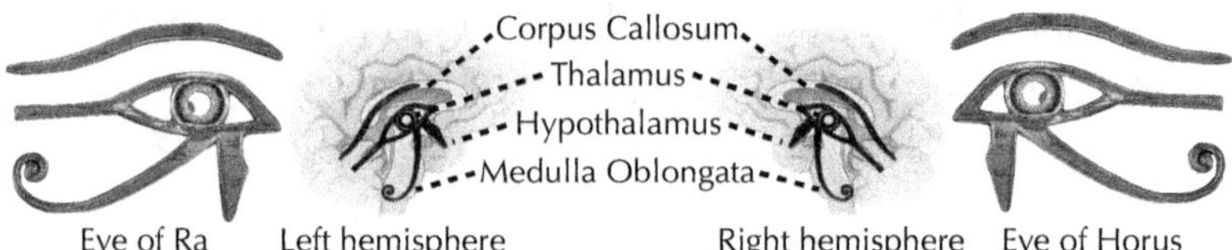

The cerebrospinal fluid flows from the ventricles to the pineal gland, which is the king, and here the spinal fluid is made electric and becomes slightly yellow in color, and is called the gold by the name of Pingala. In the pituitary gland the cerebrospinal fluid is made magnetic and becomes white in color and is called milk by the name of Idia. Now there are two different types of cerebrospinal fluid, one electrical called electro, and one magnetic, and together they become electro+magnetism, the same force that drives all electronics today; a plus and a minus, a positive and a negative, a masculine and a feminine. Plus and minus charged cerebrospinal fluid now flows out into all nerve pathways and makes the parts of the body electric and alive, therefore the world tree is also called the tree of life, which in Norse mythology is called Yggdrasil.

YGGDRASIL

The word Yggdrasil can be translated directly to "Odin's horse" and the Cauda Equina in the spine is Latin for "the horse's tail", a term the researchers of the human anatomy of the past called it, because the spinal fluid channel of the spine ends in the Cauda Equina, and then the cerebrospinal fluid continues down the nerves to the coccyx and the legs, and it looks like a horse's tail.

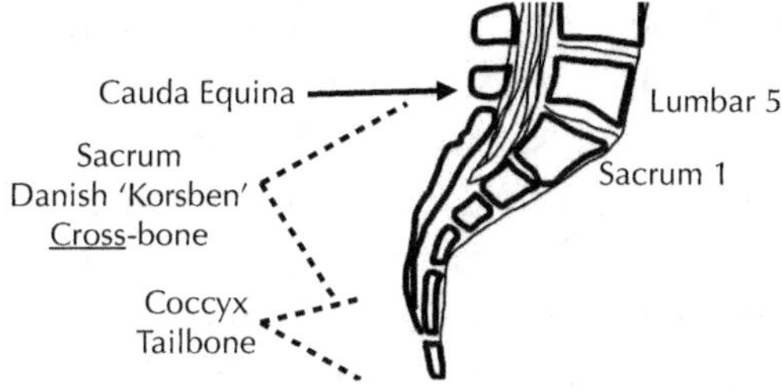

Ygg (from Ygg-drasil) is interpreted to simply mean "Odin", and at the same time the word Ygg means "the cruel". Odin has a long list of names he has called himself on his long journey through the world. One of those names is Gangleri which means a man who walks the streets, i.e. someone who wanders just as Odin is also a wanderer. The word Gangleri also means Ganglion, which is the oldest known name for nerve cells inside a nerve pathway. Nerve cells transmit electromagnetic signals throughout the body's nervous system, therefore Odin is those signals, and they come from one's thalamus, which is controlled by oneself. All people are their own Odin, who is the king of the gods, and thus a person is his own god, and the body is the horse you, as Odin himself, ride on in the outer world.

THE TREE OF KNOWLEDGE

Details about the tree of knowledge can be described as that one's knowledge is something you learn, i.e. something that you attract, and it is via. the senses. The tree of knowledge thus consists of the magnetic part of the nervous system called Idia, a female name because women represent the feminine which is the attractive negative magnetic darkness. The ventricles of the brain are called gods, and their fluid flows past the pineal gland called Joseph, and past the pituitary gland Maria, and together they form a living product of plus and minus, masculine and feminine. An electric bulb lights up when it is connected to an electric plus and a magnetic minus, and therefore the product is called the light, the sun by the name of Jesus, or in Norse mythology Baldr, who is the light of the gods.

THE FIRST AND HIDDEN SKULL

In the uterus, after the sperm and egg have joined together, a neural tube forms, a micro-small factory that begins to build the embryo. The first thing to be built is the lower part of the spine called the coccyx, the tailbone. The coccyx has four vertebrae, and on the second vertebra the first brain is formed, the Ganglion Impar, which is a small nerve sac of approximately 0.5 cm^2, from which the two first-created nerves emerge, which form the first part of the sympathetic nervous system, which is the source to thoughts of flight or attack.

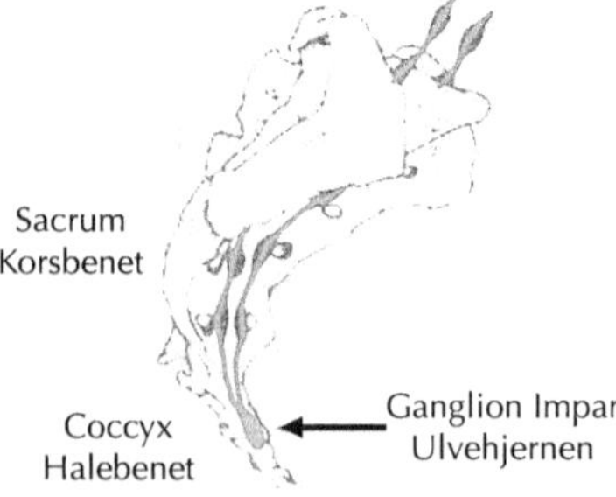

The little brain on the coccyx is a person's deepest egoistic thoughts, and is therefore called one's wolf mind, one's animal mind which is only designed to keep one alive at all costs. The coccyx has four fused vertebrae and is joined to the sacrum called the "cross bone" in Danish which has five fused vertebrae that at the bottom have two downwards bones that look like a wolf's teeth in the upper mouth.

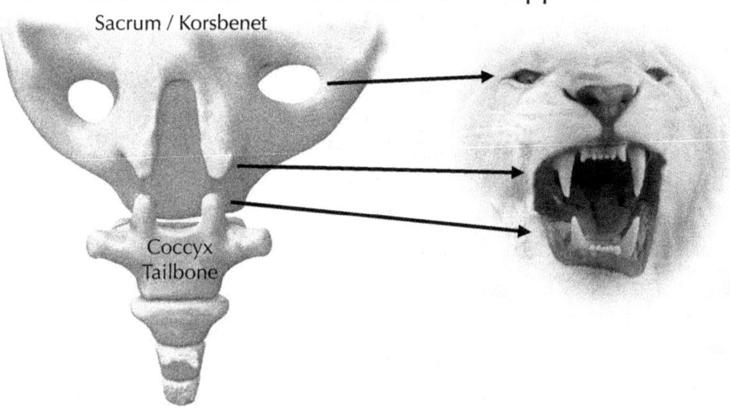

The upward "horns" of coccyx has been the inspiration for the design of countless fables and images of demons with horns on their foreheads that people fear to meet. In reality, fabled devils are just creative images of the body's inner skull consisting of the sacrum-coccyx. which symbolize one's deepest egoism, evil, anger, hatred and destruction.

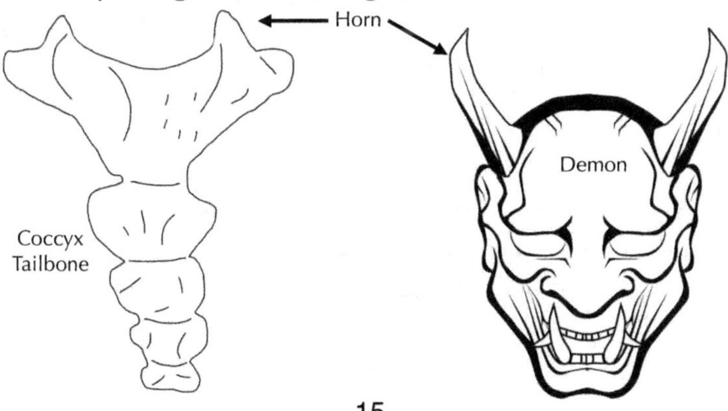

The sacrum also has four holes on each side, and a total of eight holes, and looks a bit like an alien from outer space.

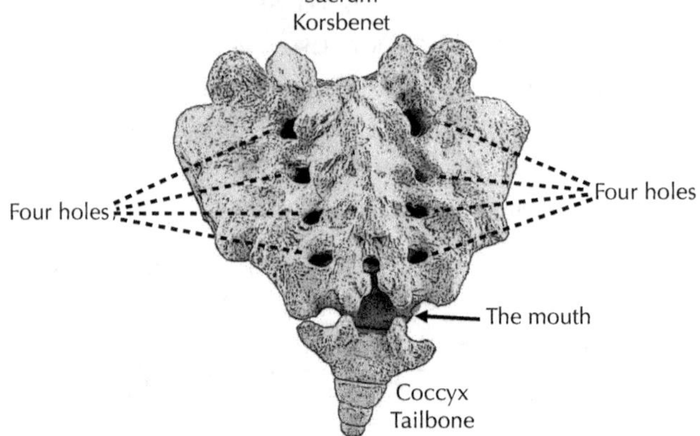

When the sacrum and coccyx are seen together, they look like an inner skull with fangs, mouth and eyes. Since the coccyx has a small real functioning brain called the Ganglion Impar, which constitutes one's deepest egoism, this skull is called one's first hidden skull that mainly seeks total control over one's entire life.

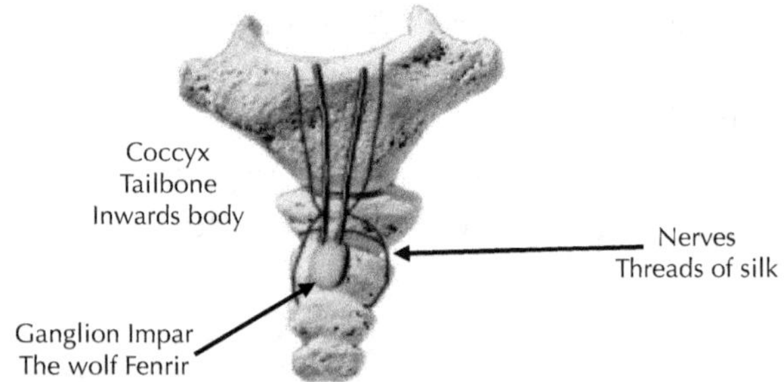

This inner skull looks like a wolf's face, and therefore in Norse mythology it is called the wolf-dog Garmr, and the wolf Fenrir, which is the brain itself located at the bottom of the second vertebra of the coccyx, and here it is bound to a stone (vertebra) with magical silk threads (nerves) around the stone. Another name for the wolf Fenrir is Vánagandr, which means "monster of the river Ván", that in Norse mythology is made of the foam from the mouth of the wolf Fenrir, because the cerebrospinal fluid flows in all nerves and looks like a river, and in this case out of the "mouth" created between the sacrum and the tailbone. The sacrum-coccyx is the great fountain named Hvergelmir which the stag Eiktyrnir's horns, the ventricles of the brain, drip cerebrospinal fluid down on where it becomes twelve rivers of nerves;

The sacrum-coccyx skull has been the inspiration for countless fantasy images of terrifying beings, all of which personify one's inner fear, anger and hatred. People who fear are easy to manipulate into anything. Countless ancient fable images and figures with horns on their foreheads are most likely misinterpreted by today's people as being real beings in a real underworld of fire where Satan lives. People tend to blindly believe in fabulous and very real fictional stories, but they are just stories, metaphors and parables. Knowledge gives you power over your own life.

MIMER'S WEL

Odin sees very well with his blind eye. Odin gave his one eye to Mimer's well to gain more knowledge and wisdom. Odin is illustrated as a man with a flap over one eye, but is has never been described which one of the eyes he sacrificed. However, Odin has a third hidden eye, just as all humans have, 'The all-seeing eye', which humans have learned to fear through through films like the one about a ring where the eye stands behind a cruel evil. Spiritually confused people have learned that the all-seeing eye is the Egyptian Eye of Ra and evil, completely unaware that this eye is their own inner third eye, the thalamus, where a person perceives everything and controls everything from, and it is Odin's eye that looks right down into Mimer's well of knowledge and wisdom. Mimer's well is under the roots of Yggdrasil (the tree of life), at the bottom of the giant Mimer's head which is the sacrum-coccyx skull. From the thalamus in the center of the third eye, in the center of the upper brain, is the body's longest cranial nerve called the Vagus nerve, which runs directly from the upper skull to the lower inner hidden skull (sacrum-coccyx) at the base of the spine. The vagus nerve is connected to all parts of the body which is the world, and therefore the vagus nerve is medically also called "the wanderer" like Odin. The vagus nerve is thus connected to Odin's third all-seeing eye in the brain of the upper skull right down to Mimer's well which is located at the Cauda Equina in the spine, from where nerves continue down to the Ganglion Impar which is the lower brain called the wolf brain which contains the first knowledge and wisdom, and one's deepest innate fears and instincts to survive in this world.

Your fear is innate, just like it is in all other humans. It is up to you to learn to know the fear and unite with it, or it will rule your entire life. The small brain on the tailbone is in occult Indian texts referred to as "The department of knowledge, and it is the wolf Fenrir called Hrodvitnir which means "famous for knowledge". Mimer's real name is Mímirsbrunnr which directly translated means "the rememberer", and memory is one's knowledge and wisdom.

Odin's inner eye is thus connected to Mímirsbrunnr, which is one's wolf brain, one's first brain on the tailbone, and from which Odin gets the deepest first knowledge and wisdom, and can thus unite with the animal knowledge and wisdom to create peace in his mind to learn new knowledge and wisdom from the outside world. When you have internal accumulated fear that has turned into anger and hatred, it is quite difficult to learn new things from the outer world, because you bite the hand of anyone who offers new knowledge, and criticism is equal to war, just as the wolf Fenrir bites the god Tyr's hand off.

<u>YOU ARE ODIN</u>

THE GREATEST INSPIRATION

About 8,000 years ago, people discovered the functions of the body, and were so fascinated that they created stories in the form of myths about it. A myth is a story so colorful, detailed and entertaining that the story told orally from person to person will be largely the same after thousands of years. Therefore, "myth-o-logies" are stories about the truth told from a supernatural point of view, through personifications and parables. Since the inner workings of the human body were the most fascinating thing about humans, all the gods, giants, good and evil beings of the great mythologies are personifications of the parts of the body. In 1918, Dr. George Carey decoded the Bible as a story about the functions of the body, and especially that Jesus and John the Baptist are personifications of the cerebrospinal fluid's journey through the body. In a detailed archaeological report of Egyptian drawings, figures and mythology, the University of California and Indiana University describe the following;

"I gather for you the gods of the north and present to you all the parts of your divine body, assembled in their place"
- 1966

I am far from the only one who has discovered similarities in the great mythologies, well-known fables and anatomical functions of the body. It may come as a shock to one that even Norse mythology with legends such as the god Odin, the demigod Thor with the hammer, the goddess Freyja and the giants are all personifications of the human body.

CRUCIFIXION

Jesus is the son of the Virgin Mary who became pregnant with God, even though she is married to Joseph. God is the Claustrum and the ventricles of the brain, which form the cerebrospinal fluid that flows to the pineal gland called Joseph, and to the pituitary gland called Mary. In the pineal gland the cerebrospinal fluid is made electric, and in the pituitary gland the cerebrospinal fluid is made magnetic, then the two different cerebrospinal fluids flow out into the nerves in each of its micro channels and create electric+magnetic known as electromagnetism, which makes the human body live and able to move. The two fluids together are the product Jesus, created by the Claustrum and the ventricles called God, the pineal gland Joseph and the pituitary gland Mary. Some texts describe that although Freyja and her brother Freyr were siblings, they were also lovers, similar to Joseph and Mary.

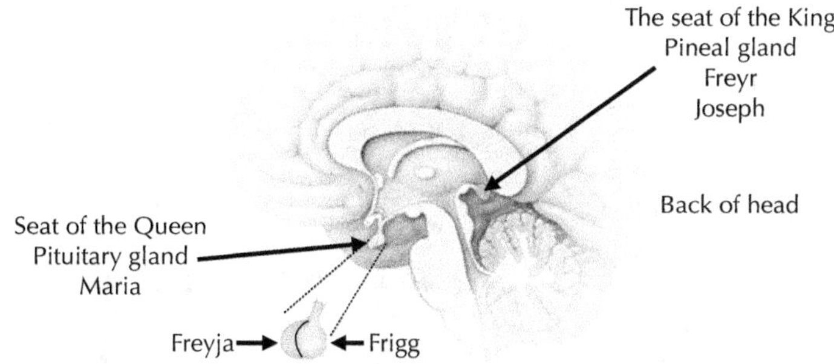

Jesus leaves the kingdom of God in the brain as a liquid and comes down to earth, the body, through the spine of 33 vertebrae, just as Jesus also became 33 years old. Jesus arrives at the Cauda Equina, the Dead Sea, which is the bottom of the spinal thecal-sac where the spinal fluid canal ends. From here Jesus travels further through nerves through the sacrum "cross bone" in Danish, and finally Jesus is nailed to the cross which is the coccyx where the sympathetic nervous system ends in the nerve sac / wolf brain Ganglion Impar. The cerebrospinal fluid called Jesus completed its journey down through the body after 33 steps of vertebrae and ended up in the Ganglion Impar nerve sac /

wolf brain which is attached to the cross which is the coccyx. In the Bible it is said that Jesus was nailed to the cross and hung there for approximately 6-7 hours, just as the cerebrospinal fluid in the body reaches its full cycle in approximately 6-7 hours. Jesus died on the cross for the sins of mankind, which means that if you live a life of fear, anger and hatred, then the cerebrospinal fluid becomes dirty and is almost dead when it reaches the small brain of the coccyx, which is fabled as if you have killed Jesus, and it can lead to pain in the abdomen and lower back because the Ganglion Impar is overstimulated due to mental inner fear that turns into anger and hatred.

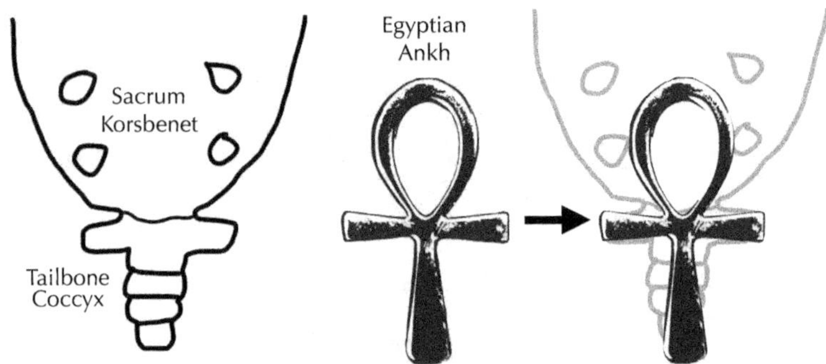

The Egyptian Ankh is known as the symbol of life, and in an archaeological report researchers describe that the Ankh is a symbol for the coccyx and the sacrum above it. Since the sacrum and coccyx are among the first parts to be created in an embryo, and the coccyx, has the first brain on it, you can say that life in a human begins, ends and is resurrected from there, just as the Ankh is a symbol of life and rebirth. The ankh is therefore the cross which i.a. is used in the biblical story of Jesus, who after the time on the cross ascended to heaven which is in the upper skull.

DRACULA

The sacrum with the coccyx also resembles Dracula's face with fangs. Dracula drinks blood because anatomical images show that the large artery above the heart branches out just above the coccyx into two arteries, one artery to each leg, and small blood vessels wind around the "mouth" of the sacrum-coccyx, so it looks like the inner skull is drinking the blood. The Mayan Blood Glyph is identified as a drawing of the lower sacrum-coccyx upside down, and from there arose the story of the lower skull drinking blood, which became Bram Stokes' fable of Dracula in the year 1897.

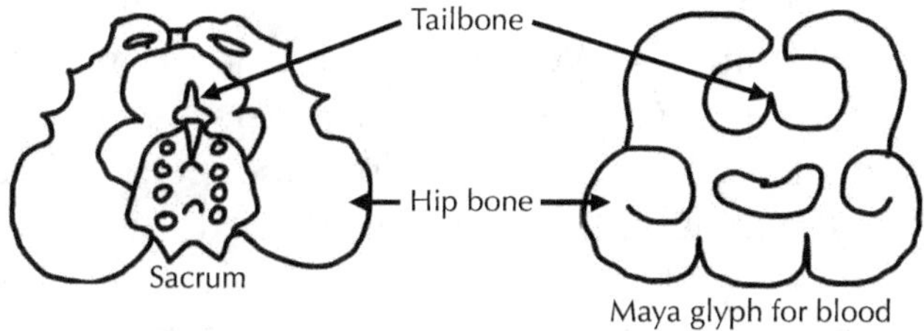

I quote Dracula's own words;

"I wasn't always Dracula, before my name was Judãhs
and I betrayed Jesus"

Dracula's own words make complete sense, because if you live a life of fear, anger and daily build up hatred for everything around you, then your life is controlled by the inner skull that has a small wolf brain that is deeply egoistic, and so makes the cerebrospinal fluid called Jesus more dirty than usual, so you can say it is betrayed. An escalating fear, anger and hatred-filled person is like Dracula and Judas who will sell his own mother for security and self-gratification, and is actually a walking dead because he is only able to live off the joy of others since he has no self-pleasure. Dracula has no mirror image because he is the inner hidden skull.

SANTA CLAUSTRUM

In the year 2020, doctors electrically stimulated an area of the brain called the Claustrum and instantly halted the person's consciousness, resulting in the person simply staring into space with the eyes open while the heart and breathing continued automatically. The experiment lasted only a few minutes. When the doctors removed the stimulation of the Claustrum in the person's brain, the person's consciousness returned, but the person had no memory of the minutes the experiment lasted. The over 200-year-old Latin word "claustrum" means "lock" or "closed place", probably because it is a place in the brain that is very difficult to examine while the person is still alive. The claustrum is located in the brain right next to the ventricles, which create the cerebrospinal fluid that flows around the entire brain and down the spinal canal, and out into all nerves in the body and back into the spinal canal and back to the upper brain. In the lower part of the spinal canal called the Cauda Equina, the spinal fluid continues down the nerves to the coccyx, where the little wolf brain is located, and here the nervous system ends and begins. The wolf brain is called Muspelheim in Norse mythology, and is the first world where everything begins and ends.

In a bar, the real Santa Claus sits in his red suit and long gray beard, drinking beer. He is a little dissatisfied and thinks the children are becoming more and more demanding and selfish every year. He gets another beer, and the bartender says to him "can you drive home after all those beers?", Santa Claus says "sure, it's the reindeer who steer the most, I only make a few adjustments along the way". The bartender looks strangely at the man who says he is Santa Claus. Santa Claus says that he was not always Santa Claus. In the past he was called Nikoerik the Red who had a hammer called Skullcrusher "Kranieknuser" in Danish. Later he became known as Weihnactsmann, which in Germanic mythology is "Julenissen" that in Danish means Father Christmas, and dolls with pointy hats were supposed to look like him. Pointy hats symbolize a person who has lifted his tailbone with the wolf brain up to the upper brain, i.e. the tailbone on top of his upper head which symbolizes that here is a wise person who is also called a magician, sorcerer and even witch, and therefore witches also have pointy hats. Later again, Santa Claus was called Saint Niklaus, who has the nickname Nikus, which is also a name for Odin in Norse mythology. Santa's name is thus connected to Niklaus and Klaus, and now remember that the area of the brain for consciousness is called Claustrum, which is personified as a man called Claus or Klaus in Danish. The first cerebrospinal fluid is thick, therefore Santa Claus is obese. The cerebrospinal fluid is made of blood, which is why Santa Claus wears red clothes. In the brain's pituitary gland, some of the spinal fluid is converted to a milky white color, and therefore Santa must also be white.

Santa with his hammer Skullcrusher sitting in a sleigh pulled by reindeer is very close to the mythological fable about Thor and his hammer, because it is the same story, Nordic mythology is just much more detailed. Even more enlightening, we can now conclude that Santa Claus is Odin, and God himself.

Santa Claus has a sleigh pulled by **eight** reindeer in the first fables. Remember that Santa, who sat in the bar and got a little drunk on beer, said that the reindeer steered the most and Santa actually just adjusted the route a little. Compare that with the fact that nerves are reins that connect the upper brain (Claustrum = Klaus = Santa Claus) with the lower part of the spine, which is the inner skull with **eight** holes that become eight reindeer in fables. Translated, it becomes Santa Claus sitting in his sleigh, which is the uppermost skull, which is pulled around the world by one's deepest egoism, which is one's lower inner skull with eight holes, which are the eight reindeer. Later, a ninth reindeer was added, Rudolf with the red nose, and the number nine became quite magical in recent times.

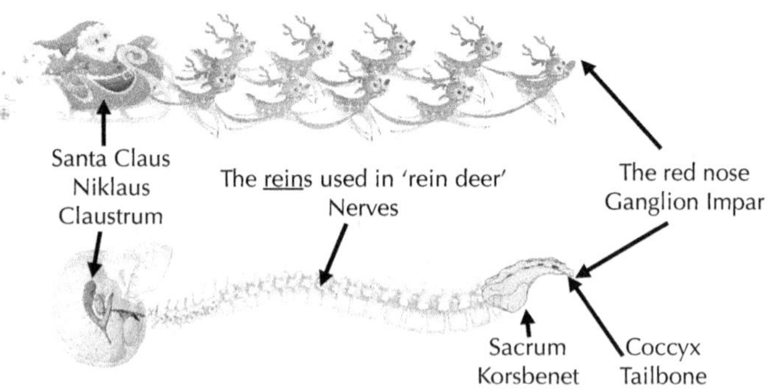

Number nine is also associated with Satanism and a world of fire, which the Bible describes as hell. The sacrum at the bottom of the spine has five fused vertebrae. The tailbone coccyx consists of four fused vertebrae. Four plus five equals nine. The sacrum has eight holes for nerves and the tailbone coccyx has the brain, Ganglion Impar, which in several languages means words like lamp and fire, and in Yoga the fire is red, so therefore the brain of the tailbone Ganglion Impar is Santa's ninth reindeer Rudolph with the red nose. Rudolf is particularly good at finding his way in very bad weather and cold, because his nose lights up and shows the way. In the most difficult moments, one is guided by one's deepest egoism, the wolf brain Ganglion Impar, to get the necessary things to get back on the feet. Those who invented and composed the fable stories about Santa Claus and the eight reindeer were later the ones to insert the ninth reindeer to include the tail bone and wolf brain in the fable.

The inner lower skull, which resembles a wolf, has led to fables about the wolf Fenrir and Dracula and can therefore be compared to the number nine, which is also described as Satan's number for perfection, which must be understood to mean that those who have united with their inner wolf brain, has full control over their own personality, which means they feel fear, anger and hatred, but see it as signals they choose to respond to or not, and that is perfection. This is what those who practice kundalini yoga seek to achieve, a union of their wolf mind and their higher mind of love and empathy. Further explained; you have to find a place for Satan in your life.

GIFTS FOR ALL IN ONE NIGHT

Santa Claus lands on the roof, which is the upper part of the spine in the head, and continues down the chimney, which is the spine, and exit over the fireplace, which is the wolf's brain on the tailbone. The wolf brain was by the Maya people called K'akh' which means fire. In India, the wolf brain is called Mula, a kind of serpent fire. In Norse mythology, the wolf brain is the world Muspelheim, a world of fire. Santa Claus is therefore the cerebrospinal fluid that flows down the spine and out of the the inner skulls mouth just above the coccyx, that is the fireplace, with gifts for the children who are one's deepest egoism that must be fed or you die. Egoism is the need for food, water, shelter, even gifts and means to keep ones body alive. The cerebrospinal fluid circulates throughout the body and is completely renewed in approximately six to seven hours. Santa Claus is the cerebrospinal fluid that delivers gifts in the form of electricity to the body so it is alive. Nerves branches out from the spine to the elements of the body and back to the spine, and this is called a "whirl" that means "world". Your body is in fables the world, and therefore Santa Claus can deliver Christmas presents to all the children all over the world in one night, or just six or seven hours.

DREAMLAND OF SANDMAN

Der Sandmann is an old German tale from the year 1800. The story in Danish is Hans Christian Andersen's fable about Ole Lukøje 'Ole Shuteye', which is inspired by the English expression "shuteye". In English you say "you look tired, you better get som shuteye", which in Danish is "du ser træt ud, du må hellere få noget <u>lukøje</u>", which clearly means sleep. Ole Lukøje or Sandman pours sand into children's eyes so they fall into sleep and dream. The English fable "The Sandman" is about a king of the dream kingdom, and he also uses magic sand to make people fall asleep and dream. We know that REM sleep is vital. REM is an abbreviation for "Rapid Eye Movement" and describes a creature that is in deep sleep and often dreams. In the year 1100, Sandman meets with a friend and overhears some young woman talking about living forever, and only one of them wants to live forever. Sandman approaches the woman and speaks only to the one who wants to live forever. The other woman leave the table, mysteriously. Now only the Sandman with his mysterious alluring confident dark appearance sits with the woman who wants to live forever.

Sandman
"you want to live forever?"

Woman
"yes"

Sandman
"I think it will drive you mind apart!"

Woman
"I can do it"

Sandman
"deal, we will meet here again in a hundred years"

Sandman leaves again, and the woman thinks this was strange. A hundred years pass and the Sandman arrives at the place as agreed, and so does the woman. The woman looks like she did a hundred years ago, no aging.

Sandman
"so, how did it go?"

Woman
"I have lost four husbands and several of my children"

Sandman
"I told you it was too hard for you"

Woman
"no, it's hard, but I have a new husband and new children"

Sandman
"so you want to continue like this?"

Woman
"yes of course"

Sandman
"We'll meet here again in a hundred years"

Another hundred years pass and the two meet again, and the eternal life continues. Thus several hundred years pass, the woman never ages, she is eternally healthy, vigorous with an youthful appearance. Who is Sandman really?, how can Sandman give the woman eternal life and eternal youth?

Sandman is a fable about a special organ in the body, namely the pineal gland in the brain. The pineal gland in the brain is medically described as being made of brain sand, i.e. sand, and if you were to personify the pineal gland in a fable, it could be a person named something with sand. The pineal gland makes the cerebrospinal fluid electric, which is an explosive positive charge and is therefore called masculine for extroverted action, and therefore the pineal gland is a 'lord', a man. In Egyptian mythology and the arrangement of pyramids, the pineal gland is the king's chamber, and the pituitary gland is the Queens chamber. A pyramid is designed like a human brain, which with the help of salty liquid can form electromagnetism. Pyramids are power plants just like a human brain is. The pineal gland is The Sandman in fables, but how can he give eternal life?

The pineal gland is the organ in the brain that produces melatonin, which flows into the cerebrospinal fluid, and further into all nerves in the body. Most people think melatonin is only a sleeping substance that makes you tired, but melatonin can heal almost any damage in the body and keep the body healthy with a youthful appearance, if you follow the rules for it. In 2014, melatonin was called the 'elixir of life' and the 'vampire hormone' by researchers because it has been found to have healing properties against virtually any ailment. In Norse mythology, the gods drink a special drink of mead that gives them eternal life, and the drink is referred to as 'the elixir of life'. In Norse mythology, the cerebrospinal fluid is mead, and the elixir of life is cerebrospinal fluid with melatonin in it. Dracula is a vampire with cold skin, and invulnerable because he heals very quickly if injured. Dracula is associated with darkness and is called the demon of darkness. Melatonin is created when the body senses darkness. Melatonin cools the body and can heal almost anything. Eg. in the case of nerve disorders or damage to the nerves, these are healed much faster than usual through light and dark therapy, which produces large nocturnal amounts of melatonin. The Sandman is a personification of the pineal gland and its melatonin that can give eternal life. The Sandman is the king of dreamland because melatonin is the reason why you sleep so deeply that you dream. The fable story of the man who was given eternal life by the Sandman is a fable that if you live and are active outside in the sunlight during the day when the Sun is above the horizon, and you are inactive and stay in total darkness or red light when the Sun is below the horizon, then you can potentially live forever. There is a lot of research into melatonin's healing properties now, even though the properties have been known for over 8,000 years, because they are described in all of the great mythologies that describe exactly how to achieve eternal life.

BIFROST

The bridge on which the gods from Asgard ride down to earth is called Bifrost that translates into 'the weak point'. We know that Asgard is the brain at the top of the world tree Yggdrasil, and we know that the earth is Midgard where people live. Midgard is everything below the brain to the 12th vertebra in the thoracic region of the spine, and the earth is the lowest parts in the thoracic region. So now we know the span of Bifrost that is the weak point and it coincides with the spine above the 12th thoracic vertebra to the top of the spine at the head being a very vulnerable area that is easily damaged by a blow, a so-called 'weak point', while a blow of the same force against the spine below the 12th thoracic vertebra will cause almost no damage, as the nerves here are protected by cerebrospinal fluid in the thecal-sac. In short, Bifrost is the nerves in the spinal canal from the upper skull and down to the middle of the spine.

ODIN TURNS INTO AN EAGLE

In Norse mythology there are nine worlds which is the whole body divided into sections called worlds. Odin is the king of all gods and he lives in Asgard which is located in the upper brain. The giants live in the lower part of the body and in particular the giants are the inner skull of the sacrum-coccyx, and the giants have the dog Garmr, the wolf Fenrir and the Midgard Serpent which, by the way, encircles the whole world, which we know is the whole body, and therefore the Midgard Serpent is the electricity in the cerebrospinal fluid and it is a serpent which in Indian fables is a serpent fire. The word 'jætte' is a Nordic word for giant, and even if people think that the fables is about real giants, it is more likely that the word giant is used for man's jætte-store (giant-sized) egoistic mind, which comes from the brain on the inner lower skull. One day, Odin is on a rampage in the deepest lands of the giants, and here he tricks a giant called Baugi into drilling a hole into a rock, after which Odin turns into a snake that crawls into the hole and steals the secret life elixir of a special mead, and then Odin transforms into an eagle that quickly flies up to Asgard with the mead where the other gods drink it. This fable is of particular importance to understand how the body works and what you can do to get this elixir of life up to your Asgard, which is your upper brain, where you will reap eternal life just like the gods. The cerebrospinal fluid is pumped around all nerves, primarily due to breathing which uses muscles that cause the cerebrospinal fluid to pump up and down in the spinal canal and around the nerves. The wolf brain on the tailbone looks like a piece of jewelry on a necklace, where the chain is two nerves from the upper spine. The cerebrospinal fluid flows most easily down the nerves to the wolf brain (Ganglion Impar), but it is more difficult to pump the cerebrospinal fluid up from there again, and therefore there is a tendency for the wolf brain to swell due to too little flow in the cerebrospinal fluid there. The giant's name 'Baugi' means 'ring-shaped' and in the body there is only one known ring-muscle, and it is the sphincter muscles whose tendons are connected to the tailbone around the area where the wolf brain (Ganglion Impar) is located. If you contract your sphincter muscles, you create pressure and flow in the cerebrospinal fluid in the wolf brain. When you inhale via the breath, the cerebrospinal fluid is pumped / vacuumed upwards towards the brain. Breath is oxygen, movement of air, and birds that fly symbolize the element of air. An eagle is one of the fastest birds that can fly at very high speeds. When Odin transforms into an eagle, it means that the breath lifts the mead upwards, and now we are directly connected to kundalini yoga from India, where one seeks to lift the wolf mind up to the upper mind. By doing such pinching exercises of the sphincter muscles, called Mula Bandha in Indian, together with strong inhalation through the nose, older cerebrospinal fluid in the wolf brain is lifted out into the spinal canal and up to the brain, which is the god Odin, with the help of the giant Baugi, that sucks stored cerebrospinal fluid out of small holes that are nerves from the wolf brain that is hidden on a mountain that is the tailbone. This practice is one of the most cleansing for the entire nervous system and especially the brain, which is cleaned of waste substances faster than usual, which leads to a higher than normal cognitive function that makes one faster to think and find creative solutions to daily challenges, which gives a much better life in all areas, and that in itself is life-prolonging.

DARKNESS AND MEDITATION

The pituitary gland is divided into two glands; the front part produces several types of hormones for eg. reproduction, mood and joy, but also growth hormones which repair the body. All these characteristics fit with the characteristics of the Norse goddess Freyja, who in the fables is very similar to the Norse goddess Frigg. Freyja is the front (closest to the forehead) part of the pituitary gland and Frigg is the back (inwards towards the midbrain) part. The god Odin is married to the goddess Frigg, but Freyja is Odin's mistress, and this coincides with the fact that doctors nowadays call the pituitary gland 'The Mistress gland'!

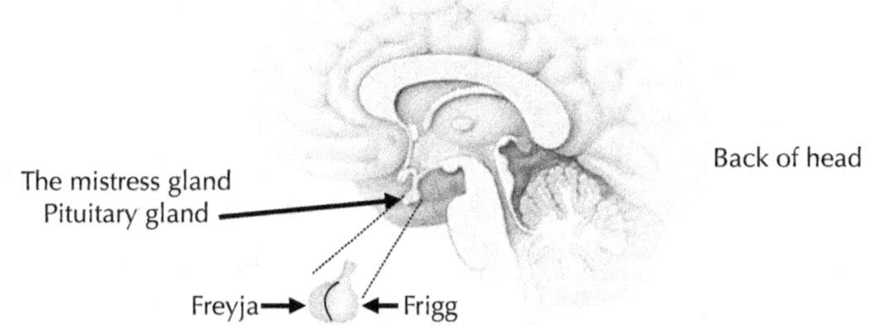

In Norse mythology, Freyja's chariot is pulled by two cats, but cats can never be enslaved. In Egyptian mythology, cats are associated with the eyes, and the mythologies tell the same stories just with different figures and different names, therefore the cats are the eyes that pull Freyja's chariot.

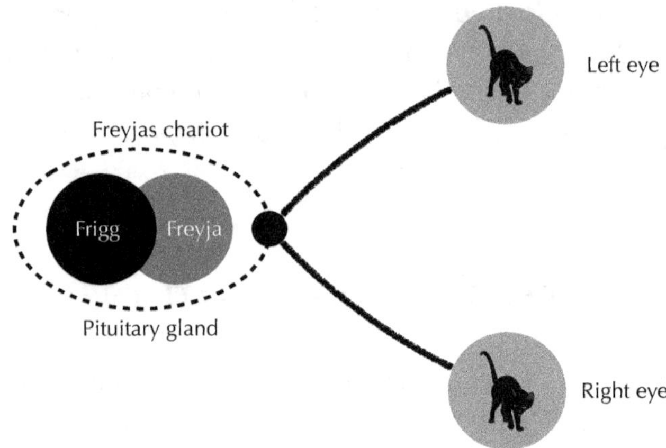

Seen from above, the two cats are the two eyes in the head and the optic nerves from the eyes are the reins to Freyja's chariot, which is the pituitary gland where the optic nerves cross right in front. Cats are feminine beings. Feminine means negatively magnetic charged which belongs to the category of silence and darkness. Studies show that people make far more health-promoting hormones and increase their reproductive hormones by up to 49% when they meditate in the dark, which is why the fable of Freyja's chariot being pulled by two cats is a fable of Freyja, the anterior part of the pituitary gland, increasing its effect significantly when the eyes are closed, and especially when you turn your 'sight' inwards and become like a cat; quiet and calm in the dark. Frigg is at the back of Freyja's carriage and is the rear part of the pituitary gland, which produces the hormone oxytocin which, among other things, increases growth and healing. The production of oxytocin is highest at night, just as cats are animals of the night because the night is feminine and dark. The dark is where thieves and some dangerous animals hunt, and then you have to protect your children, and Frigg is the great mother who also produces hormones vasopressin that increases emotions that increase vigilance and necessary behavior to protect the family and territory. The old fables are truly stories about the functions of the body, and the fables are gifts to mankind, if only people understood the true meaning of the fables. Unfortunately, the vast majority of people are blind to unpacking metaphors and fable stories, so instead they cultivate the personifications in the fable stories or turn them into religion, where it rarely leads to the real life-prolonging properties, which the Bible paradoxically describes itself; Those who take these words (of the Bible) literally will die. Those who understand that the words are parables and live by them will find eternal life!

SATAN 666 THE DEVIL

Humans has been taught to fear Satanism like the dark. The Book of Revelation describes that the number 666 is the number of man. It is the human body and man's inner wolf mind of pure egoism, driven by fear, anger and hatred that is the devil named Satan with the number of the beast 666, not a devil with horns who rules in a real world of flames where the souls of naughty people are thrown into. Being a Satanist means that you take care of your body, get the necessary food, warmth and comfort so it lives optimally, and this is smart because it is only your body that is the ticket to live physically in this world. The upper mind of love and empathy must be nurtured as much as one's body. One's upper evolved wolf of love and empathy must be fed as much as one's lower inner wolf of egoism. Connecting the upper mind with the lower mind is what Egyptian mythology calls raising the Djed-pillar, lifting the lower wolf mind up to the high evolved mind and uniting them. As long as you can do that you are a Djed, which means stability or balance. The Egyptian Djed column has four rings that resembles the four vertebrae on the coccyx. In Norse mythology, the balance is described by lifting the Midgard Serpent up to the sky, with the fable of the god Thor who is enticed to show his strength in the land of giants, where the Midgard Serpent is disguised as a particularly long and large cat. Thor almost lift the cat so high that one of its paws is lifted off the floor. Everyone in the hall becomes afraid, because if Thor lifted the cat all the way up to heaven it would change the laws and the entire structure of the world. After only 60 days of Kundalini yoga, it can scientifically measured that one's DNA and genes are altered, and the body is the whole world in Norse mythology! Thor's home has 640 rooms and the human body has 640 muscles. Thor is a personification of i.a. the body's muscles, that must be used to breathe strongly inwards while contracting the sphincter muscles to lift the cerebrospinal fluid and its charge (The Midgard Serpent) from the Ganglion Impar upwards to heaven which is in the mind in the upper brain. What the Bible describe as God, and what Nordic, Egyptian and Sumerian mythology tells is the Gods are something inside yourself. You are your own God or Gods. You are your own Osiris, Odin or Shiva while your inner ego is Horus, the giants or Shakti. Some people believe in religion so literally that they wait for their savior to arrive the second time and save everything and pay all the bills for them. They are going to wait until they have killed themselves in ignorance. All saviors are personifications of the cerebrospinal fluid, and it is totally renewed every 6-7 hours or so, so everyone is sort of saved every 6-7 hours. When you are filled with fear, anger and hatred, you breathe incorrectly, and breathing is the primary function of the cycle of the cerebrospinal fluid, which now flows too slowly around the body's nervous system, and in the upper brain it leads to more than normal amounts of waste products that decreases one's cognitive abilities leading to slower reaction in the mind. In the lower brain, it causes an abnormal pressure that is signaled as pain in the abdomen and lower back, and thoughts of fear that turn into anger and hatred increase. Intelligence decreases and one's immune system weakens. In short, you are in the process of killing yourself. The cerebrospinal fluid contains special white blood cells which are part of the immune system, and removes the waste products of the body's elements. The many billions of small parts of the body work constantly, and can be compared to a car with the engine running in a closed garage. Without cleansing the toxic substances such as e.g. carbon monoxide, even the engine will suffocate due to lack of oxygen, and it is the same in the body. The body's elements must have a constant supply of nutrients and oxygen to function, and they must constantly have waste products removed that otherwise turn into acid that breaks down tissue, a destructive condition known as cancer. A completely clean and well pumped around the body cerebrospinal fluid can keep a person healthy forever, which was described by doctors in 1917.

YOGA

Kundalini yoga is a great way to pump the cerebrospinal fluid more than usual around the whole body, to promote the whole nervous system which is the brain. Kundalini yoga uses contraction of the sphincter muscles along with the necessary special breathing techniques. The Fenrir wolf brain Ganglion Impar is constantly growing from accumulated fear, anger, hatred and cerebrospinal fluid, and therefore it must have a release, e.g. with this selected technique;

1. Preferably stand up, or sit down as another choice
2. Exhale the air from the lungs
3. Contract the sphincter muscles
4. Inhale deeply through the nose and hold your breath
5. Pull the abdomen up under the ribs and hold it there as long as it is comfortable to hold the breath
6. Release the sphincter muscles
7. Exhale through the nose, preferably with a little pressure

Optionally, raise the arms above the head when inhaling, and lower the arms again when exhaling. Do this exercise three times in a row a day and it's already a great start.

LIGHT AND DARK THERAPY

The pineal gland, is also medically described as a magnetosensor, that can sense electromagnetism. This world consists of 12 hours of light when the Sun is above the horizon, and 12 hours of darkness when the Sun is below the horizon. When the Sun is above the horizon, it is the domain of light and the entire electromagnetic field above the earth's surface changes. The pineal gland perceives whether it is day or night, regardless of eyesight. During the day, production of melatonin is minimized or halted. During this period, the body is expected to receive sunlight and form the hormone-like substance vitamin D. In the domain of the light, the body expects low levels of melatonin. Vitamin D and melatonin counteract each other. When the Sun is below the horizon, it is the domain of darkness, and the pineal gland wants to produce melatonin, but only if the eyes and body are in darkness. Sufficient amounts of melatonin can only be produced if there are sufficient amounts of vitamin D in the body. When seeking eternal life one must cultivate the domain of darkness which is dark surroundings and silence, and one must sleep in total darkness and silence. The ear canals can lead light into the pineal gland and disrupt the production of melatonin, and that's one reason why some monks wear a hat that has flaps that cover the ears. People seek health and healing in the domain of light, which is eg. noise and physical activity. The way of the light can heal very little compared to the way of darkness. The light can only save the soul while the body die of aging and disease. Humans are awake far too long with artificial light far into the domain of darkness. They sleep with their electronic devices that light up brightly at night. When the body senses light for just a moment in the domain of darkness, it can delay the production of melatonin for up to two hours. Without the correct amount of melatonin in the body in the domain of darkness, disorders begin in the body. Diabetes and cancer are first on the list of ailments caused by lack of sleep and melatonin. Medically published studies show that, among other diseases, diabetes and cancer show strong decline when cultivating light and dark therapy.

DARK MEDITATION

Jesus says that those who have gone into themselves can find eternal life. Going into yourself is as simple as closing your eyes, and it is the simplest form of meditation. Before bed every night in your totally dark bedroom;

1. Sit on the edge of the bed
2. Close your eyes
3. Breathe correctly with the stomach at the navel, deeply in and out, quietly and calmly
4. Think of your thoughts as serpents that bite you if you give them attention or stare at them for too long. You will lose any battle against your thoughts, so let your thoughts flow freely. Instead, count your breaths to keep your focus there
5. Fold your hands in your lap
6. Sit like this for 33 minutes

Go straight to bed and sleep afterwards. You must not look at any light sources for the 33 minutes and until you wake up again. The above method is one of the most healing methods known in the world, because it will stimulate high natural and acceptable amounts of the highly healing melatonin from the pineal gland directly into the cerebrospinal fluid which is pumped around well with your correct breathing with the navel / stomach. Melatonin gets around in the smallest parts of your entire body most of the dark night, and now we're talking properties that only the Sandman can give you.

DARKNESS KNOWS EVERYTHING

When you are active, extroverted and think long and hard to find solutions to problems and challenges, you are in the domain of the light, that has very little knowledge and wisdom, and a lot of noise so you use your life energy and age, become sick and dying. Darkness is the mother who is also called the father because it can give you something, because it created everything that exists and it constantly receives magnetic information from all living things and the experiences of all living things. The darkness contains all knowledge and all wisdom in all worlds everywhere, inside and outside, above and below. You must seek and cultivate the darkness if you want access to the totally superior library of all knowledge and wisdom. You have to look to the dark when you are looking for answers and solutions. You do this by making yourself completely calm, being quiet, close your eyes and just be, breathe deeply and very slowly. Soon the darkness will find you and you it, and knowledge and wisdom will be shared with you so you can solve any problem, any challenge with the highest creativity which is ingenuity. You must befriend the father and mother of darkness, whom you have probably learned to fear from those who want to keep your knowledge and wisdom at a slave level.

Once a very skilled knight asked the Dark Emperor;

The knight
"What can you give me?"

Emperor of Darkness
"EVERYTHING"

DJED

Both the light and the dark are ultimate forces that are deadly and will kill you if you are too close to one, and too far away from the other. You must seek to live in 50% light and 50% darkness every day, then you will become the most balanced being you can be, and in Egyptian mythology this is called a Djed. Your weapon as Djed is illumination, a sword of light, a sword of enlightenment which is such wise words that you can win over a thousand soldiers with them.

SAMSON AND THE LONG HAIR

Samson was a man of God and had long hair just like Jesus who was also a man of God. A man represents the masculine, and long hair is a feminine quality. A man with long hair symbolizes a man in perfect balance of the light masculine and the dark feminine. Samson won over a thousand soldiers with the jawbone of a donkey. A donkey is a top-class wise animal, and jawbone means that Samson speaks such wise words with his own jawbone of a mouth that he can overcome the minds of a thousand soldiers with his words. You as a Djed, like Samson, can win over any situation with your smarter than normal knowledge and wise mind. You become so confident you become invincible, you become a Djed.

TO SELL ONE'S SOUL TO SATAN

The mythical figure Satan knows your deepest personality completely. Movies where people have sold their souls to Satan for success and wealth is a fable that those who cultivate the darkness at the right times achieve great success and wealth because all the answers to success and wealth are found in the darkness. Satan is just a mythical figure representing darkness. Talking too much costs one's focus so it is difficult to achieve one's goals. Wait to speak until the darkness has wisely formulated just the right often few words of wisdom in your mind. This can only be achieved through patience and silence while the darkness works in your mind. Through the practice of this you will soon discover how quickly the darkness can compose perfect words of harmony in your mind, and others will soon respect the beautiful wise symphony of words you utter, and you. Speaking is the domain of light, extroverted masculine action. Listening is the domain of darkness, introverted feminine action. Most are out of balance to either the dark side or the light side. Talk as much as you listen. Spend the same amount of time performing actions as you spend having your eyes closed and being inside yourself. If you want to know yourself you must find Satan within yourself.

DARKNESS AND LIGHT

To observe the magnetic attraction of a cat to a dog is like observing the game between the magnetic attraction of darkness to light. Darkness is silent and has all wisdom. The light is noisy and has almost no wisdom. The dog (the light) often lacks wisdom and runs too fast to the cat (the darkness) only to be met with a slap or worse from the cat and the dog howls loudly as the wisdom is burned into its memory about cats through the pain in the nose. The light and the dark seek to cancel each other out constantly and it is the essence of life that also tells you to keep your nose to yourself, because if you stick it too far into other people's affairs you will get a slap. Mind your own business in your own home, keep your critical opinions about other people's homes to yourself.

HUGINN & MUNINN

In Norse mythology, the god Odin has two ravens he uses to spy on everything in the world. Instead of wandering out to spy himself, Odin can send two ravens. The two ravens are known throughout the human outer common world as Huginn and Muninn. The name Huginn means thought. Muninn means memory, so it is now logical how Odin gets information from the world, the body, with the help of the two ravens, where he receives the information in his inner all-seeing third eye which is now illuminated with information. This is why we say "I see" = "eye see" and means that one's inner all-seeing eye which is you, your essence, your soul sees = understands. Huginn and Muninn are both associated with goddesses who determine one's happiness, wealth and success in life, and this is true. If your mind lives mostly in the dead past of bad memories, you will slowly kill yourself this way. Think of a freshly cut slice of lemon in your mouth and you feel your mouth water just because of the thought. Think of a delicious piece of food and soon you will be hungry because the body's stomach changes the stomach acid and prepares the intestines for more food, just because of the thought. Think of something bad in the past and feel where in the body discomfort arises. This is due to changes in blood pressure, heart rate and changes in hormones to tune the body to what you are thinking about, the past, that the body thinks is happening right now. Thinking about the past too often and for too long will kill you in the long run. Memory must be used as experience and wisdom about how to be in the present. If you send Muninn the raven flying all the time in your memory, it will get exhausted, fall down and die. If your thoughts are constantly in motion and you don't give your body and thoughts a break, Huginn the raven will fly until it is exhausted, fall down and die. The three Norns Urd, Skuld and Verdani at the bottom of Yggdrasil spin your destiny and determine your age. Their names mean Past, Present and Future. The holiest Norn is Urd who is the past, your well of wisdom. You yourself are the three Norns who spin your own destiny that determines how long you live, with the choice of which wells you use the most.

THORS HAMMER

The solar plexus controls eg. the function of the lungs, the breath. Thor's hammer Mjölner is constructed by the dwarves Sindri and Brokkr. The dwarf Sindri's name is close to the

Danish word "sind" that means "the mind", thoughts and willpower. Sindri also means "the spark" that is electromagnetic signals in the nerves, and a thought is electromagnetic. Brokkr controls the bellows that blows air to the fire when Thor's hammer Mjölnir is constructed. Without the hammer, Thor is almost powerless in battle, and this makes sense, because without the willpower of the mind Sindri and Brokkr to control the bellows that are the lungs of the human body, no muscles will get any oxygen to be able to move. Thor's hammer Mjölnir is what gives a man his strength to do anything. Mjölnir always hits the target it is thrown at, just like in an argument or battle with another creature, the wrath in that scenario always hits the creature it is aimed at. Mjölnir always returns to Thor after it is thrown. Mjölner is used almost exclusively to hit someone in the head with, hence the hammer's older name Kranieknuser / Skullcrusher. When the hammer Mjølner / Skullcrusher is thrown at someone, it mostly hits them in the head, after which the hammer returns to Thor who often has to wear an iron glove to protect himself from the force of the hammer. Angry words from your mouth to another's brain which is in a skull, can crush the other's skull which is their mind, and the result can be a hard 'blow' back at you. The word hammer is from the word Hamarr, meaning 'a hard rock or stone', so being hit by a hammer from Thor is like being hit by a rock. Thor's deadly lightning and thunderbolts are words in the form of curses from the mouth that strike those they are aimed at. Gnostics describe how evil words from one person to another can harm a person's mind so that the person's life becomes mentally deteriorated and sad inside, from the evil words often leading to illness and early death of the person. Thor's lightning and thunder are also interpreted as your own thoughts judging you, which shortens your own life, as the word hammer is referred to as God or the hammer of the gods that can kill you, and God and the gods are yourself. The personification of Hamarr is the demigod Thor who is also known by the name Düvel which means death or devil, just as the biblical texts describe; that the beastly man is the devil himself. The devil is also referred to as the beast. Book of Revelation 13:18;

"This calls for wisdom. Let the person who has insight calculate the number of the beast, for it is the number of a man. That number is 666."

BALDR & THE MISTLETOE

Baldr has a dream where he is killed, so his mother the goddess Frigg, makes him invulnerable to everything on earth, except the mistletoe, which grows in a high place far from Valhalla. The gods play with Baldr, throwing weapons, stones and things at him, but he cannot be hurt, he is protected by the magic of Frigg. Strangely, Frigg tells an old lady who is Loki in disguise that only the mistletoe can harm Baldr. Loki quickly gets hold of the mistletoe and, according to some texts, turns the mistletoe into an arrow and tricks the blind god Höðr into shooting the arrow at Baldr. The arrow kills Baldr and everyone is sad. The name of the blind god is Höðr, meaning "warrior", "war", "slaughter", "battle". This blind god is described in some texts as a god of the underworld from a world of darkness where no sight is useful, therefore he is blind. Baldr's name means 'shining', and he is referred to as 'the shining one', he is also the light of the gods. In some old texts, Baldr is described as a sky god who brings light, just as Jesus is also God's light. The mistletoe as the only weapon that can kill Baldr is a metaphor, because commonly known mistletoe is a plant that can cure many diseases and increase fertility. The mistletoe is best known for hanging over doorways and if two people stand under the mistletoe they must kiss and therefore the mistletoe represents the idea of kisses leading to blind love and thoughts of sex, and the sexual arousal that happens in the body when it thinks on sex, or having sex leads to signals in the body's hormones that reproduction has taken place, and in fact, deeper studies show that sex with the opposite sex shortens the life of both partners, a result that has also been observed in mealworm beetles. The mealworm beetles that refrained from reproduction lived significantly longer than those that did reproduce. When one becomes sexually excited, a gate called 'the fish gate' opens at the 12th thoracic vertebra of the spine, and the small store of cerebrospinal fluid in the Solar Plexus leaks out into the cerebrospinal fluid in the spine, and now the person loses the stored buffer of electromagnetically charged cerebrospinal fluid to the muscles and often feels weak in the legs, and it shortens one's lifespan if it happens too often. Religious priests and nuns must refrain from sex and from being sexually excited. In short, Baldr can be thought of as the stored buffer of electromagnetically charged cerebrospinal fluid in the Solar Plexus, and therefore the mistletoe can kill him because it often leads to thoughts of sex. In a collected modern version about Baldr, it is the goddess Hel who is tired of living in Helheim, the world of the dead. Helheim is the lower part of the sacrum bone where nerves look like grids down to the brain of the coccyx, the world of fire Muspelheim. Helheim is a metaphor for people who live so selfishly without any kind of empathy for others that Gnostics call them 'walking deads', i.e. walking dead egoistic people. Such a condition is also called 'a living death for the soul'. The goddess Hel of Helheim contacts Loki and makes a plan so that Hel can bring Baldr down to her. Loki kills Baldr with the mistletoe and Baldr descends to the goddess Hel. Baldr tells Hel jokes about Asgard and Hel laughs so loudly and happily that the whole of Helheim lights up with joy, because Baldr is the light. The story is a metaphor that if you succumb to your own egoism when it comes to sex, your life of egoism will feel great right now and probably for a long time, but it costs the eternal life of the body, which will age, get sick and die. If you live a life of egoism and no empathy for other living beings, you live in Helheim, <u>the world of the dying</u>, and it will kill your body.

CLAIRVOYANCE & SEJD

Freyja and Frigg are magicians who performs an art called 'seidr' or sejd, and if you listen to the word sejd, it sounds almost like 'sight'. Sejd is the visualization of the inner third all-seeing eye because the pituitary gland is Freyja and Frigg. Odin also uses the art of sejd to see the future. The pituitary gland is responsible for the inner creation of vision from the two eyes, but also the creation of visualization from visions and hallucinations. A highly active and developed pituitary gland can provide the experience of flashes of light emerging from within the brain when receiving psychic visions, also called spiritual clairvoyance. If there is alcohol in the body it can cause disordered functioning of the pituitary gland and this can create false illusions of the eyes, vision and hallucinations. If there is a lot of alcohol in the body and you are heavily intoxicated, the pituitary gland can almost become paralyzed, and this is the reason why seers, practitioners of sejd and clairvoyance are forbidden to drink alcohol. The pituitary gland is only one part of the entire inner all-seeing eye, which also includes the pineal gland. The more you practice your inner all-seeing third eye, the more vivid your inner vision becomes, and you can even have visions while the two outer eyes are open. Visions of landscapes, places, people will arise and soon you will be able to see much more, and this art is called sejd in Norse mythology. The art of Sejd can get its information directly from the cerebrospinal fluid, which is highly conductive to electrical and magnetic energy. All living organisms everywhere, emit electromagnetic signals from their cerebrospinal fluid and nerve cell activity, which contain thoughts and visions, and all this information is sent out into the great cosmos of everything, the air, the water, the earth. You can simply ask your inner all-seeing third eye what you are looking for and it will begin to show you what you are looking for, even with sound or voices, because the third inner eye is also a third inner ear.

RAGNARÖK & FENRIR

The wolf Fenrir's parents are Loki and Angrboða. Loki is an unpredictable trickster, and Angrboða means 'one who brings or offer grief" or even 'one who brings harm'. The first word Angr means anger. These traits create a wolf with a mind that is easily angered and causes harm. The gods fear the wolf Fenrir, so they trick him into seeing how strong he is by tying him to a rock, but he is only willing to do so if a god puts his hand in the wolfs mouth. The brave god Tyr puts his hand in the mouth of the wolf Fenrir. The very special chain the gods have made is called Gleipnir, and is as thin as silk threads and stronger than any chain. The wolf Fenrir cannot break free from the chain, so he is now tied to the stone, and he bites Tyr's hand. After this Tyr was nicknamed 'the remains of the wolf', meaning that the wolf only ate Tyr's hand and left Tyr with the rest of his body. This action shows that the wolf Fenrir is something that harms others when anger arises. In a phenomenon called ragnarok, the wolf Fenrir will break free from the chain and swallow the god Odin, and this leads to the death of the wolf Fenrir and Odin, which is a metaphor for uniting the lower wolf mind with the highest developed empathic mind, creating a new perfect mind. Ragnarok is war and electromagnetic mixing of the thoughts in the lower wolf mind of pure egoism with the upper mind of love, understanding and empathy, exactly like the Indian concept of kundalini, which is achieved by lifting one's wolf mind up to the upper mind through pinching exercises of the anus and breathing techniques. I call the techniques Ragnarök Jöga, which leads to one balanced mind, and one becomes an Egyptian Djed master.

FAITH CAN MOVE MOUNTAINS

In published medical studies, it is described that the brain is internally controlled by words. If a person has heard of e.g. the Nordic demigod Thor and his abilities, it becomes words and visions in the person's mind, which in this way commands the body and mind to have the same powers as Thor, and this is measurably enhancing the person's abilities. Every human being has the god power to do anything and all it takes is a strong belief and inspiration from the gigantic perfectly constructed fables and myths of mankind. People have healed themselves with strong faith that the gods or just a single god healed them. When a single organ in the body is personified, one's thoughts can be targeted with electromagnetic thought commands to that organ seeking to do as dictated, as doctors in 1940 proved. Dampening or strengthening an organ in the manipulative way can weaken other organs and <u>you can injure yourself</u>, therefore such a practice requires a great anatomical knowledge of the body.

FABLES AND MYTHOLOGY TO YOU

Many have told me over time that I live in a fantasy world, but so does everyone else. Many town names in Norway and Sweden, several road names and places in Denmark are named after Norse mythology. In the high north of the body are the three kingdoms of the brain consisting of the creator gods Høj, Jævnhøj and Tredje. In the northern part of the Earth is Scandinavia with its three kingdoms. Perhaps that is why Denmark is a leading country in this world. Any device was first an idea, and then build.

From an Island of Enlightenment I Santa Claus brought the unwrapped gifts from the mythologies and fables to you. Use them diligently and achieve the highest with yourself.

See you again in a few hundred years